PREGNANCY WORKOUT GUIDE:

Safe and Effective Workout

for Every Pregnant Woman

Dr. Vera J. Reynolds

ACKNOWLEDGEMENT

I would like to take a moment to acknowledge my parents, Francis and Mary, who have been a constant source of support and inspiration throughout my life. My father, a dedicated medical doctor, instilled in me a deep appreciation for the importance of health and wellness. His knowledge and expertise have been invaluable in the creation of this book, and I am forever grateful for his guidance.

My mother, Mary, has always been my biggest cheerleader and has encouraged me to pursue my passions and follow my dreams. Her unwavering support and love have given me the confidence to tackle any challenge, including the creation of this pregnancy workout guide.

To both of my parents, I say thank you from the bottom of my heart. Your love, guidance, and encouragement have shaped me into the person I am today, and I am honored to dedicate this book to you.

TABLE OF CONTENTS

CHAPTER ONE

INTRODUCTION

Annie had always been an energetic individual. She enjoyed jogging, weightlifting, and attending exercise courses. So, when she found out she was

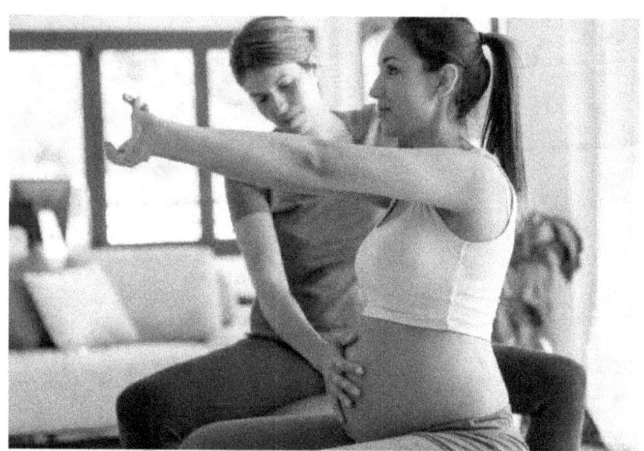

pregnant, she was determined to maintain her athletic lifestyle. However, Annie needed clarification about what activities suited her and her developing infant. She wanted to remain healthy and robust throughout her pregnancy but didn't want to put herself or her infant in danger.

Annie knew she required direction, so she looked

to her psychiatrist for counsel. Her doctor recommended a maternity exercise program to help her remain fit while assuring her safety and the baby. Annie was enthusiastic about the concept but was also apprehensive. She had heard conflicting reports about exercising during pregnancy and didn't want to take any chances.

Still, Annie resolved to give the maternity exercise guidance an opportunity. She grabbed a book and started reading. The handbook covered everything she needed about exercising during pregnancy, from the advantages of keeping active to the exercises safe for expecting mothers.

Annie was delighted to find out that exercise could genuinely assist her throughout her pregnancy. It could decrease the chance of gestational diabetes, hypertension, and other pregnancy-related complications. Plus, it could help her maintain a healthy weight and prepare her body for childbearing.

The maternity exercise handbook also described the different safe routines for expecting mothers. Annie discovered that cardiopulmonary activities, such as strolling and swimming, were excellent for maintaining general fitness and could be done throughout her pregnancy. Strength training activities, such as bodyweight movements and small weights, could help her maintain muscle density and support her expanding abdomen. The guidance also included exercises and yoga postures that could help her remain flexible and alleviate discomfort.

Annie was surprised by how comprehensive the maternity exercise program was. It even included information on nourishment and hydration, caution signals to watch out for, and modifications for typical pregnancy conditions. She felt confident she had all the skills needed to maintain a healthy and lively pregnancy.

Annie started incorporating the movements and stretches from the handbook into her daily regimen. She observed an immediate improvement in her energy levels and general well-being. She also appreciated the modifications for typical pregnancy complaints, such as sickness and back pain, which helped her remain comfortable throughout her exercises.

As Annie's pregnancy progressed, she followed the maternity exercise guidance. She appreciated the attention to safety and the explicit instructions for each practice. She felt powerful and competent, knowing she was caring for her body and her infant.

Finally, the day arrived, and Annie gave birth to a thriving newborn daughter. She felt thankful for the maternity exercise guidance, which helped her remain healthy and active throughout her pregnancy. She understood that she would continue to use the advice to help her recuperate and reclaim her vitality postoperatively.

Annie's experience testified to the significance of keeping active during pregnancy. With the proper instruction and preparations, expecting mothers can maintain their exercise levels and enhance their general health. The maternity exercise guide was invaluable for Annie and could be for any prospective mother seeking to remain fit and healthy throughout her pregnancy.

Pregnancy is a period of tremendous transformation for a woman's body. With the developing infant, changing hormones, and an enlarging uterus, it's comprehensible that many women may feel reluctant or uncertain about continuing to exercise during this time. However, remaining active during pregnancy has numerous advantages for both mother and infant, including enhanced cardiovascular health, decreased chance of gestational diabetes and hypertension, and better mental health.

The Pregnancy Workout Guide is intended to provide women with a comprehensive reference for safe and efficient exercise during pregnancy. This guidance is designed to be a beneficial tool for women of all exercise levels and phases of pregnancy, whether you're a seasoned athlete or just beginning out. The handbook contains information on safe exercise during pregnancy, modifications for typical pregnancy complaints, and exercise safety considerations.

The first trimester can be particularly challenging for many women, who may experience exhaustion, sickness, and other pregnancy symptoms. However, it's still essential to remain moving during this period. The guidance includes various safe activities during the first trimester, including cardiovascular exercises like strolling and stationary pedaling, strength training exercises that use body weight or light weights, and stretching and yoga exercises to promote flexibility and relaxation.

As you progress into the second trimester, your body will continue transforming and adjusting to the developing infant. The guidance suggests modifications for typical pregnancy complaints during this period, including back discomfort, puffiness, and shortness of breath. It also contains safe and beneficial activities for developing strength and maintaining cardiovascular health during the second trimester.

In the third trimester, your body will experience even more alterations as it prepares for childbirth. The guidance includes safe activities during this time and modifications for typical pregnancy complaints like abdominal discomfort and difficulty relaxing. It also provides information on actions that can help prepare your body for labor and delivery.

After childbearing, many women may feel uncertain about how to securely and successfully restart the exercise. The handbook contains information on certain postpartum activities and when it's safe to begin exercising after childbirth. It also provides instruction on progressively increasing the intensity and duration of exercise over time.

In addition to providing exercise recommendations, the Pregnancy fitness Guide also contains information on proper nourishment and hydration during pregnancy and how to choose appropriate fitness attire. It also provides essential safety considerations for exercising during pregnancy, including warning signals to cease exercising and protections for high-risk pregnancies.

Overall, the Pregnancy Workout Guide is a comprehensive resource for women wanting to remain active and healthy during pregnancy. Following the recommendations and modifications outlined in this guide can improve your physical and emotional health during pregnancy, prepare your body for childbirth, and establish a foundation for lifetime health and well-being.

Benefits of exercising during pregnancy

Exercising during pregnancy has numerous advantages for the mother and the developing child. Here are some of the most significant benefits:

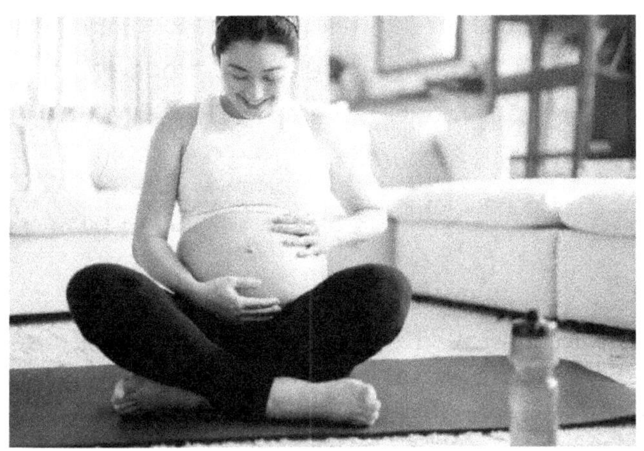

- **Improved general health and fitness:** Exercise during pregnancy can help improve cardiovascular fitness, physical strength, and endurance, as well as enhance overall health.

- **Reduced risk of gestational diabetes:** Regular exercise during pregnancy has been shown to reduce the risk of gestational diabetes, a form of diabetes that happens during pregnancy.

- **Reduced chance of preeclampsia:** Preeclampsia is a condition that can develop during pregnancy and is distinguished by elevated blood pressure and protein in the urine. Regular exercise has been shown to decrease the chance of preeclampsia.

- **Improved weight management:** Exercise during pregnancy can help women control their weight and prevent excessive weight growth, which can contribute to complications such as gestational diabetes and premature delivery.

- **Reduced risk of cesarean delivery:** Regular exercise during pregnancy has been shown to lessen the risk of cesarean delivery.

- **Improved mood and decreased stress:** Exercise has been shown to improve mood, reduce stress, and diminish symptoms of melancholy and anxiety during pregnancy.

- **Improved sleep quality:** Exercise can enhance sleep quality during pregnancy, essential for general health and well-being.

- **Preparation for labor and delivery:** Exercise can help prepare the body for labor and delivery by increasing strength, endurance, and flexibility.

It is essential to remember that pregnant women should communicate with their healthcare practitioner before beginning any exercise program and observe their recommendations for safe and efficient exercise during pregnancy.

Safety considerations

Safety considerations are essential when it comes to practice during pregnancy. Here are some important safety considerations to bear in mind:

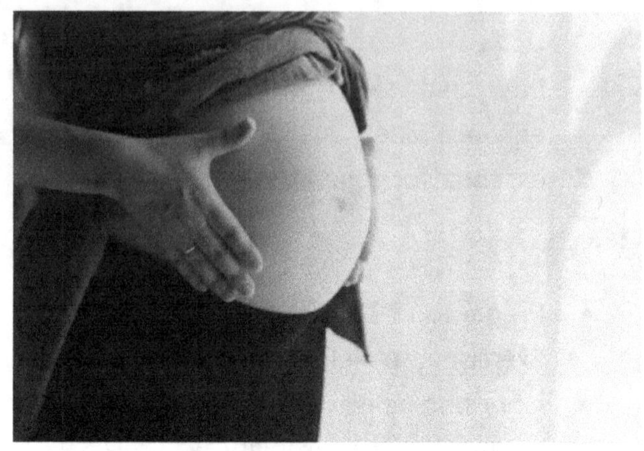

- **Please discuss this with your healthcare provider:** Before beginning any exercise program during pregnancy, it is essential to consult with your healthcare provider to ensure that it is healthy for you and your developing child.

- **Listen to your body:** During pregnancy, your body experiences significant changes, and it is essential to listen to your body and prevent any activity that causes pain, discomfort, or exhaustion.

- **Avoid certain kinds of exercise:** Pregnant

women should avoid high-impact and collision sports and any activity with a risk of tripping or abdominal injury.

* **Stay moistened:** It is essential to stay moisturized during activity, particularly during pregnancy drink liquids before, during, and after exercise.

- **Avoid hyperthermia:** Pregnant women should avoid overheating during exercise, as it can be hazardous for the developing child. Avoid practicing in sweltering and steamy conditions, and wear loose-fitting, breathable clothing.

- **Adjust exercise as needed:** As your pregnancy progresses, you may need to adjust your exercise regimen to accommodate your shifting body. This may include decreasing the intensity of your exercises or transitioning to lower-impact practice.

- **Avoid laying flat on your back:** After the first trimester, pregnant women should avoid lying flat on their back for prolonged durations, as it can diminish blood supply to the cervix.

- **Pace yourself:** Exercise moderately and pace yourself during your exercise. Avoid straining yourself too hard or attempting to increase your power or endurance rapidly.

By observing these safety considerations, pregnant women can exercise securely and experience the many advantages of physical activity during pregnancy.

How to use this guidance

This maternity fitness guide provides information and advice on exercising securely and successfully during pregnancy. Here are some suggestions on how to use this guide:

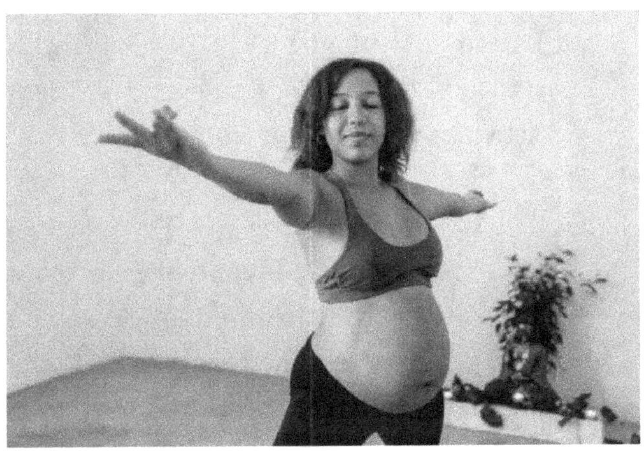

1.   **Read through the guide:** Start by perusing the complete guide to familiarize yourself with the information and suggestions supplied.

2.   **Discuss with your healthcare provider:** Before beginning any exercise program, it is essential to consult with your healthcare provider to ensure that it is healthy for you and your developing child.

3.   **Choose safe and appropriate activities**: Choose exercises that are safe and appropriate for your fitness level and period of pregnancy. The handbook provides instances of safe and efficient activities for pregnant women.

4.   **Start gently and eventually increase intensity:** Start with low-intensity exercise and progressively increase the intensity and frequency of your activities over time.

5.   **Listen to your body:** Listening to your body and preventing any activity that produces pain, irritation, or exhaustion is essential. If you experience any caution indications during exercise, cease immediately and communicate with your healthcare practitioner.

6.   **Adjust activities as needed:** As your pregnancy progresses, you may need to change your exercise regimen to

accommodate your shifting body. The handbook provides suggestions on adjusting activities for each period of childbearing.

7. **Stay moistened and well-nourished:** It is essential to stay refreshed and well-nourished during pregnancy, particularly during activity. Drink plenty of water before, during, and after training, and maintain a healthy and balanced diet.

By following these guidelines and using the information in this guide, you can securely and successfully incorporate exercise into your maternity regimen and experience the many advantages of physical activity during pregnancy.

CHAPTER TWO

First Trimester Workouts

Many women experience exhaustion, sickness, and other early pregnancy symptoms during the first trimester of pregnancy. However, frequent exercise during this trimester can help increase energy levels, reduce tension, and prepare your body for the physical challenges of pregnancy and childbirth.

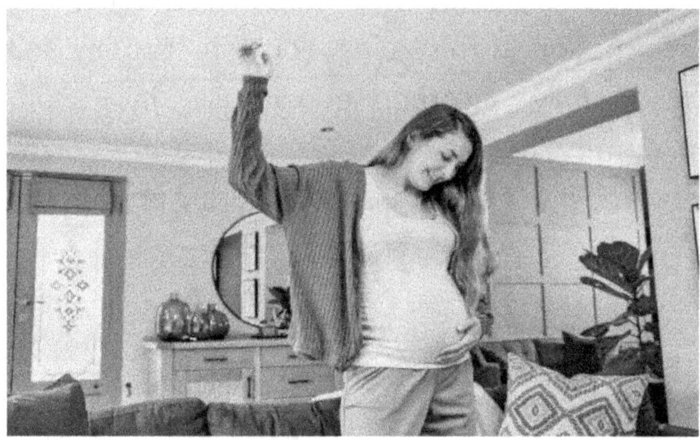

It's essential to remember that your body is going through many changes during the first trimester, so it's vital to modify your exercise regimen appropriately. This may mean decreasing the intensity and duration of your routines and concentrating on delicate low-impact movements on your joints.

In this portion of the program, we will examine different fitness choices that are safe and efficient during the first trimester, including cardiovascular activities such as strolling and swimming, as well as strength training exercises that can help maintain muscle tone and prevent damage. It's essential to consult with your healthcare practitioner before beginning any exercise regimen during pregnancy, listen to your body, and make modifications as required.

Cardiovascular activities

Cardiovascular exercise is an essential component of any fitness program, and it can be securely and successfully incorporated into a maternity training regimen. Here are some safe and efficient cardiovascular activities for pregnant women:

Walking:

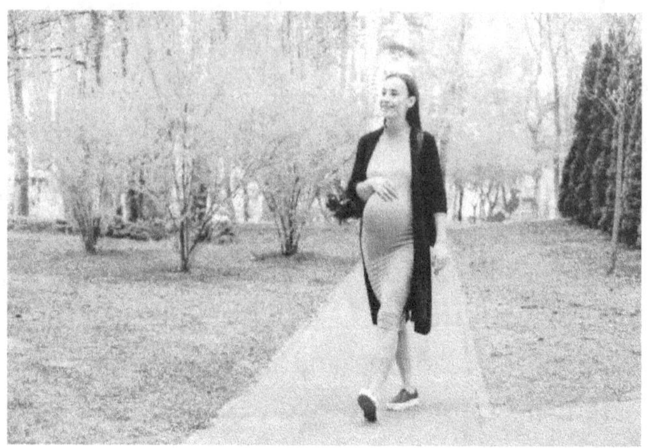

Walking is a secure and low-impact activity that can provide numerous health advantages for pregnant women. Here are some suggestions for safe and efficient strolling during pregnancy:

1. **Wear comfortable and supportive shoes:** Invest in decent strolling shoes that provide support and cushioning. Your ankles may expand during pregnancy, so choose sandals with additional space.

2. **Start leisurely and gradually increase the duration and intensity:** Begin with brief treks and progressively increase the duration and intensity over time. Aim for 30 minutes of exercise daily, most days of the week.

3. **Choose secure and even surfaces:** Stick to level, even emerge free from obstructions and dangers. Avoid strolling on slippery or irregular surfaces.

4. **Use good balance:** Maintain excellent posture while strolling. Keep your shoulders relaxed, your head horizontal to the ground, and your abdominal muscles engaged.

5. **Stay moistened:** Drink plenty of water before, during, and after your stroll to stay hydrated.

6. **Avoid overheating:** Avoid strolling during the warmest portion of the day and remain in protected places or indoors when feasible. Wear loose-fitting, breathable garments.

7. **Listen to your body:** Avoid pain, irritation, or exhaustion while strolling. Slow down or pause if necessary, and communicate with your healthcare practitioner if you experience any concerning symptoms.

Walking can provide numerous health advantages during pregnancy, including enhanced cardiovascular health, increased energy levels, and decreased tension and anxiety. It is essential to consult your healthcare practitioner before beginning any exercise regimen and observe their recommendations for safe and efficient exercise during pregnancy.

Swimming:

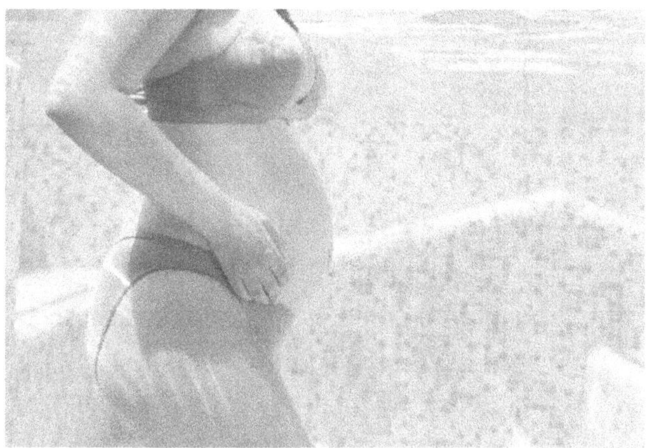

Swimming is an excellent low-impact activity that can provide numerous health advantages for pregnant women. Here are some guidelines for fast and efficient swimming during pregnancy:

- **Choose a secure environment:** Swim in a safe, well-maintained pool free from dangers and obstructions. Make sure the water is clear and adequately purified.

- **Start leisurely and progressively increase intensity:** Begin with shorter swimming practices and gradually increase the endurance and power over time. Aim for 30 minutes of swimming daily, most days of the week.

- **Use excellent technique:** Use the correct swimming technique to prevent pressure on your body. Avoid excessively exhausting strikes or movements.

- **Keep moistened:** Drink plenty of water before, during, and after swimming to keep refreshed.

- **Wear appropriate swimwear:** Wear a well-fitting, comfortable swimsuit that provides support and covering.

- **Avoid overheating:** Avoid swimming for prolonged amounts of time or in uncomfortably heated water. Take pauses and relax when required.

- **Listen to your body:** Pay attention to any pain, irritation, or exhaustion while swimming. Slow down or pause if necessary, and communicate with your healthcare practitioner if you experience any concerning symptoms.

Swimming can provide numerous health advantages during pregnancy, including enhanced cardiovascular health, increased muscular strength and flexibility, and decreased tension and anxiety. It is essential to consult your healthcare practitioner before beginning any exercise regimen and observe their recommendations for safe and efficient exercise during pregnancy.

Stationary cycling:

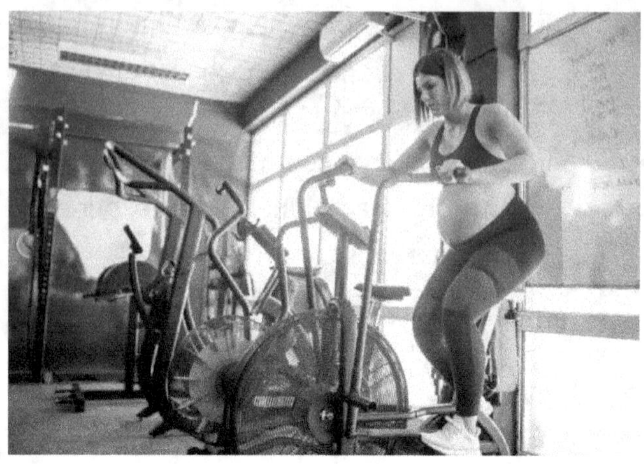

Stationary pedalling is a low-impact activity providing numerous health advantages for pregnant women. Here are some guidelines for safe and efficient static pedalling during pregnancy:

1. **Adjust the cycle to your comfort level:** Make sure the saddle height and handlebar location are modified to your comfort level. Your knees should be slightly bowed when the wheels are at their lowest position.

2. **Start leisurely and progressively increase intensity:** Begin with shorter pedalling workouts and gradually increase the endurance and power over time. Aim for 30 minutes of pedalling daily, most days of the week.

3. **Use good balance:** Maintain excellent alignment while pedalling. Keep your shoulders relaxed, your head horizontal to the ground, and your abdominal muscles engaged.

4. **Avoid standing on the pedals:** Avoid standing on the pedals, as this can increase the risk of accidents or damage.

5. **Keep moistened:** Drink plenty of water before, during, and after pedalling to stay hydrated.

6. **Wear appropriate clothing:** Wear

comfortable and breathable clothing that provides the flexibility of movement.

7.   **Listen to your body:** Avoid pain, irritation, or exhaustion while pedalling. Slow down or pause if necessary, and communicate with your healthcare practitioner if you experience any concerning symptoms.

Stationary pedalling can provide numerous health advantages during pregnancy, including enhanced cardiovascular health, increased muscular strength and flexibility, and decreased tension and anxiety. It is essential to consult your healthcare practitioner before beginning any exercise regimen and observe their recommendations for safe and efficient exercise during pregnancy.

Elliptical trainer:

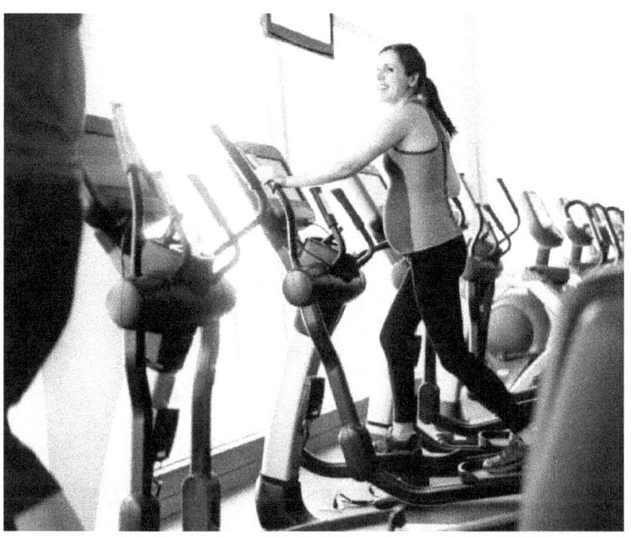

The elliptical trainer is a low-impact exercise equipment that can provide excellent training for pregnant women. Here are some guidelines for the safe and efficient use of the elliptical machine during pregnancy:

1. **Adjust the machine to your comfort level:** Make sure the stride duration and difficulty level is modified to your comfort level. Start with a modest resistance setting and progressively increase the

intensity over time.

2.   **Start leisurely and progressively increase intensity:** Begin with shorter exercises and gradually increase the endurance and power over time. Aim for 30 minutes of elliptical exercise daily, most days of the week.

3.   **Use good posture:** Maintain excellent alignment using the elliptical machine. Keep your shoulders relaxed, your head horizontal to the ground, and your abdominal muscles engaged.

4.   **Avoid using equipment with moving arms:** Some elliptical trainers have movable arm controls. Avoid using these handles during pregnancy, as they can increase the risk of accidents or injury.

5.   **Stay hydrated:** Drink plenty of water

before, during, and after using the elliptical machine to stay refreshed.

6. **Wear appropriate clothing:** Wear comfortable and breathable clothing that provides the flexibility of movement.

7. **Listen to your body:** Pay attention to any pain, irritation, or exhaustion while using the elliptical machine. Slow down or pause if necessary, and communicate with your healthcare practitioner if you experience any concerning symptoms.

The elliptical machine can provide numerous health advantages during pregnancy, including enhanced cardiovascular health, increased muscular strength and flexibility, and decreased tension and anxiety. It is essential to consult your healthcare practitioner before beginning any exercise regimen and observe their recommendations for safe and efficient exercise during pregnancy.

Aerobics classes:

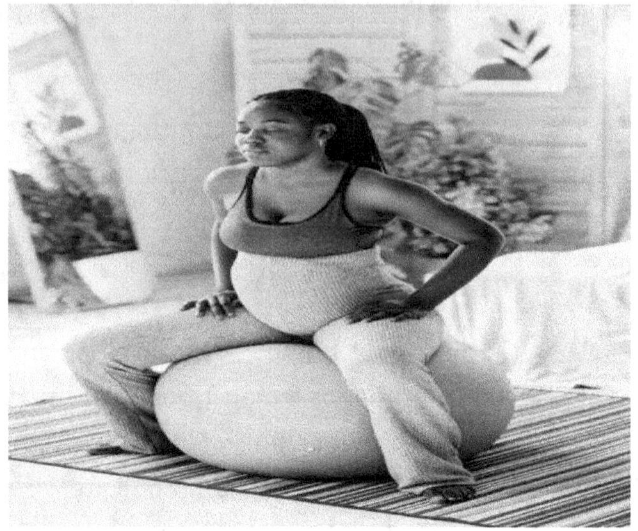

Aerobics lessons can be a fantastic way to remain active and healthy during pregnancy. Here are some guidelines for safe and successful participation in exercise courses during pregnancy:

1. **Choose a low-impact class:** Look for a low-impact exercise session for pregnant women. High-impact activities, such as leaping and sprinting, can place too much stress on your joints and increase the

chance of damage.

2.   **Check with your healthcare provider:** Before beginning any exercise program, consult your healthcare provider to ensure it is secure for you and your infant.

3.   **Inform the instructor:** Tell the instructor you are expecting, and ask for modifications or substitute activities as required.

4.   **Keep moistened:** Drink plenty of water before, during, and after the exercise to stay refreshed.

5.   **Wear appropriate clothing:** Wear comfortable and breathable clothing that provides the flexibility of movement.

6.   **Use excellent technique:** Use correct

technique and posture to prevent pressure on your body. Avoid excessively strenuous activities or calisthenics.

7. **Listen to your body**: Pay attention to any pain, difficulty, or exhaustion during the session. Slow down or pause if necessary, and communicate with your healthcare practitioner if you experience any concerning symptoms.

Exercise lessons can provide numerous health advantages during pregnancy, including enhanced cardiovascular health, increased muscular strength and flexibility, and decreased tension and anxiety. It is essential to consult your healthcare practitioner before beginning any exercise regimen and observe their recommendations for safe and efficient exercise during pregnancy.

Dancing:

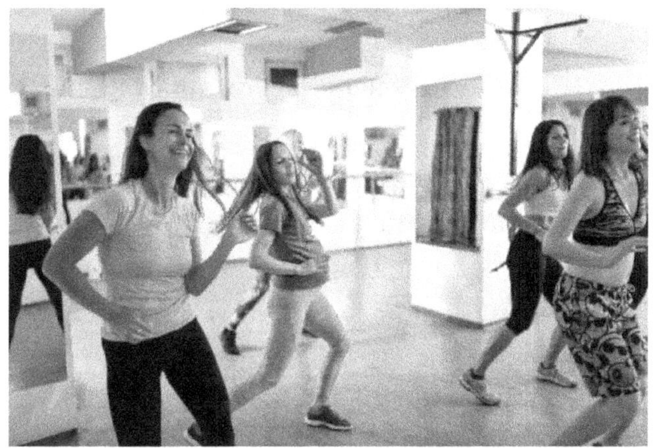

Dancing can be a pleasant and pleasurable

way to remain active and healthy during pregnancy. Here are some guidelines for secure and efficient dancing during pregnancy:

1. **Choose low-impact dances:** Look for low-impact dance techniques for pregnant women, such as ballroom or Latin dancing. Avoid high-impact dance techniques, such as hip-hop or tap dancing, which can place too much stress on your joints and increase the risk of injury.

2. **Check with your healthcare provider:** Before beginning any ballet lessons, consult your healthcare provider to ensure it is secure for you and your infant.

3. **Inform the instructor:** Tell the ballet instructor you are expecting, and ask for modifications or substitute movements as required.

4. **Use excellent technique:** Use correct technique and posture to prevent pressure on your body. Avoid excessively strenuous activities or callisthenics.

5. **Stay moistened**: Drink plenty of water before, during, and after exercising to stay hydrated.

6. **Wear appropriate clothing:** Wear comfortable and breathable clothing that provides the flexibility of movement.

7.   **Listen to your body**: Pay attention to any pain, difficulty, or exhaustion during dancing. Slow down or pause if necessary, and communicate with your healthcare practitioner if you experience any concerning symptoms.

Dancing can provide numerous health advantages during pregnancy, including enhanced cardiovascular health, increased muscular strength and flexibility, and decreased tension and anxiety. It is essential to consult your healthcare practitioner before beginning any exercise regimen and observe their recommendations for safe and efficient exercise during pregnancy.

Interval training:

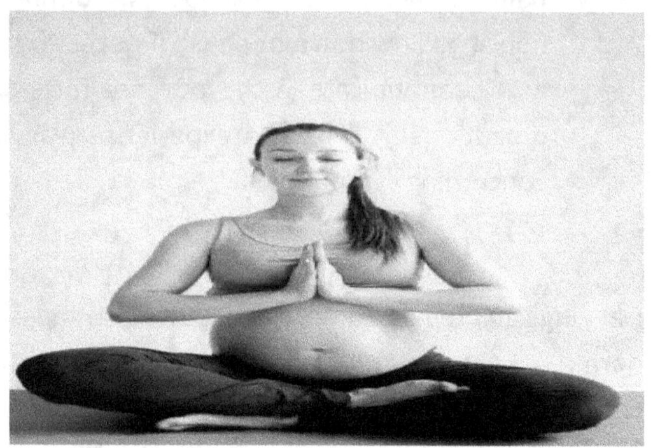

Interval training is a form of cardiovascular exercise alternating between high-intensity spurts and moments of relaxation or low-intensity exercise. Here are some suggestions for safe and efficient interval exercise during pregnancy:

1. **Check with your healthcare provider:** Before beginning any endurance exercise program, consult your healthcare provider to ensure it is safe for you and your infant.

2. **Start leisurely and progressively**

increase intensity: Begin with shorter repetitions and gradually increase the endurance and power over time. Aim for no more than 20-30 minutes of intense exercise daily, most days of the week.

3. **Choose low-impact activities**: Select low-impact exercises, such as strolling, cycling, or swimming, to minimize the chance of damage.

4. **Monitor your heart rate:** Keep watch of your heart rate during endurance exercise to ensure it does not surpass the recommended target range for pregnancy (typically 140-150 beats per minute).

5. **Stay hydrated:** Drink plenty of water before, during, and after endurance exercise to stay refreshed.

6. **Use good posture and technique:**

Maintain good posture and technique while practicing to prevent pressure on your body. Avoid excessively strenuous activities or callisthenics.

7. **Listen to your body:** Pay attention to any pain, irritation, or exhaustion during endurance exercise. Slow down or pause if necessary, and communicate with your healthcare practitioner if you experience any concerning symptoms.

Interval exercise can provide numerous health advantages during pregnancy, including enhanced cardiovascular health, increased muscular strength and flexibility, and decreased tension and anxiety. It is essential to consult your healthcare practitioner before beginning any exercise regimen and observe their recommendations for safe and efficient exercise during pregnancy.

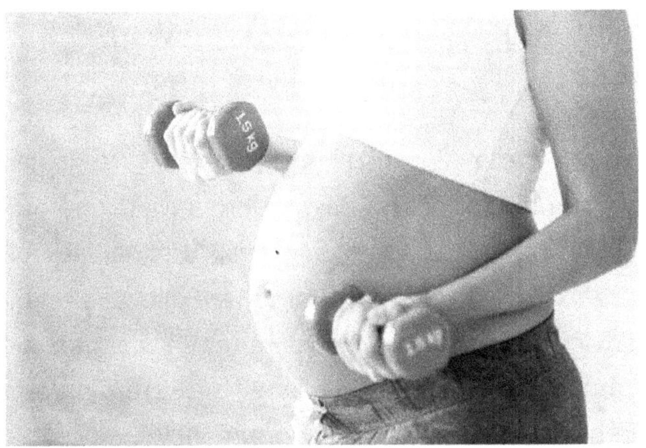

Strength training during pregnancy can help you preserve muscular mass, decrease the chance of gestational diabetes and hypertension, and enhance your general strength and fitness. Here are some suggestions for safe and efficient physical exercise during pregnancy:

Check with your healthcare provider:

Checking with your healthcare practitioner before beginning any exercise program during pregnancy is crucial to ensure your safety and the welfare of your infant. Your healthcare practitioner can evaluate your medical background and present health condition to prescribe safe and appropriate exercise choices.

They may also provide particular recommendations or restrictions based on your circumstances, such as high-risk pregnancies or pre-existing medical conditions. Following their advice can help you avoid potential dangers or complications and achieve the tremendous benefits of exercise during pregnancy.

It is also essential to keep your healthcare practitioner notified of any changes in your exercise regimen or if you experience any difficulty or complications while exercising during pregnancy. This can help them observe your health and make any necessary modifications to your exercise routine.

In summation, conferring with your healthcare practitioner before beginning any exercise program during pregnancy is vital for ensuring your safety and your infant's safety. They can provide individualized recommendations and instructions to help you accomplish a secure and prosperous exercise regimen during pregnancy.

Choose appropriate weights:

Choosing appropriate weights during pregnancy is essential to prevent damage or pressure on your body. It's vital to consider your present fitness level and period of gestation when selecting consequences for strength training activities. Here are some suggestions for choosing appropriate weights during pregnancy:

1. **Start with light weights:** If you are new to strength training, start with small weights or just your body weight. Gradually increase the weight or resistance as your strength and endurance increase.

2. **Use moderate weights:** If you have experience with strength training, strive

for middling consequences that you can raise for numerous repetitions. Avoid carrying large weights that may cause fatigue or damage.

3. **Adjust your weights as your pregnancy progresses**: As your pregnancy progresses, your body may require weight modification. Listen to your body and decrease the weight or intensity of your movements if you experience any difficulty or pain.

4. **Consider resistance bands:** Resistance bands can provide a secure and efficient alternative to conventional weights during pregnancy. They offer customizable resistance and can be used for a variety of activities.

5. **Focus on proper form and technique**: Regardless of your weight or resistance, good condition and style are crucial to

preventing damage or fatigue. Make sure you are using the correct form and technique during each practice.

In summation, selecting appropriate weights during pregnancy is essential for preventing damage or strain. Start with small weights and progressively increase the weight or resistance over time. Listen to your body and modify your weight as your pregnancy progresses. Focus on correct form and technique during each activity to prevent injury or fatigue.

Use correct technique and form:

Using correct technique and form during strength training activities is essential for minimizing damage and assuring the effectiveness of your practice. Here are some suggestions for using the right method and posture during pregnancy:

1. **Maintain correct alignment:** Stand or recline with proper balance throughout the activity. Keep your spine straight and shoulders relaxed.

2.   **Engage your core:** Engage your core muscles to support your vertebrae and maintain equilibrium during the activity.

3.   **Keep your movements gradual and controlled:** Avoid abrupt or unexpected activities that can cause fatigue or damage. Keep your actions gradual and maintained throughout the practice.

4.   **Don't retain your breath**: Remember to breathe during the activity. Exhale during the exertion portion of the movement and breathe during the relaxation phase.

5.   **Avoid activities that put pressure on your midsection:** Avoid exercises that require you to lay on your back or put too much pressure on your abdomen, such as crunches or sit-ups.

6. **Use appropriate grasp and foot placement:** Use the proper grip and positioning for each practice. This can help you maintain correct posture and technique and prevent damage.

7. **Start with smaller weights:** Start with lighter weights and concentrate on the correct form and technique before progressively increasing the weight or resistance.

In summation, using correct technique and form during strength training activities can help prevent damage and guarantee the effectiveness of your practice. Focus on maintaining proper alignment and activating your core, keep your movements gradual and controlled, remember to breathe, avoid activities that put pressure on your midsection, use the correct grasp and foot positioning, and start with smaller weights.

Incorporate bodyweight exercises:

Incorporating bodyweight movements during pregnancy is a beautiful way to increase strength and flexibility without needing apparatus or additional weight. Here are some bodyweight movements that you can incorporate into your maternity fitness routine:

1. **Squats:** Squats are an excellent lower body activity that can help strengthen your thighs and buttocks. To execute a squat, stand with your feet shoulder-width apart, activate your core, and gently lower your body down as if you were reclining in a chair. Ensure your ankles remain behind your heels and your spine stays straight. Return to the beginning position and repeat for several repetitions.

2. Lunges are another lower body activity that can help increase strength and balance. To execute a lunge, commence with your feet hip-width apart, move one foot forward and lower both knees, maintaining you're back straight. Return

to the beginning position and continue on the other side.

3.   **Push-ups:** Push-ups are an excellent upper-body activity that can help strengthen your torso, arms, and shoulders. To execute a push-up, commence horizontally with your palms shoulder-width apart and your ankles together. Lower your torso to the ground, keeping your forearms close to your sides. Push back up to the beginning position and repeat for several repetitions.

4.   **Planks:** Planks are excellent practice for strengthening abdominal muscles. Start horizontally with your palms shoulder-width apart and your ankles together. Hold the position for 30 seconds to a minute, concentrating on activating your abdominal muscles.

5.   **Bridges:** Bridges are excellent practice

for strengthening your buttocks and lower back muscles. Start by laying on your back with your knees bowed and your feet level on the ground. Lift your pelvis towards the ceiling, tightening your buttocks at the peak of the exercise. Lower your pelvis back down and continue for several repetitions.

Incorporating callisthenics movements during pregnancy is an excellent method to increase strength and flexibility without needing apparatus or additional weight. Some bodyweight movements to attempt include squats, lunges, push-ups, planks, and bridges. Make sure to concentrate on correct form and technique during each practice to prevent damage.

Take pauses as needed:

During pregnancy, it's essential to listen to your body and take pauses as required during your exercise regimen. Here are some suggestions for getting breaks during maternity workouts:

1. **Rest when needed:** If you feel exhausted or lethargic during your exercise, pause and rest. This will enable your body to recuperate and minimize the chance of damage.

2. **Hydrate:** Make sure to remain refreshed during your activity by consuming water before, during, and after exercise. Dehydration can contribute to lethargy and other health concerns.

3. **Adjust the workout:** If you discover that a particular exercise is too challenging or creates difficulty, modify the activity or transition to a reduced-intensity practice. For example, you could change push-ups by completing them on your knees instead of your heels.

4. **Take numerous pauses:** If you conduct a lengthier exercise, take frequent breaks to relax and recuperate. This will help you maintain your energy levels and minimize

the danger of overexertion.

5. **Listen to your body:** The essential thing is to listen to your body and take pauses as required. If you feel uncomfortable or experience discomfort, halt the activity and relax.

In summation, having pauses as required during pregnancy exercises is essential for remaining secure and healthy. Rest when needed, stay hydrated, adjust the training appropriately, take numerous delays, and listen to your body. By following these measures, you can maintain a secure and efficient exercise regimen throughout your pregnancy.

Stay hydrated:

Staying moisturized during pregnancy is essential for both you and your developing infant. When you exercise, your body sheds fluids through sweat, and it's necessary to replenish them to prevent dehydration. Here are some suggestions for keeping refreshed during maternity workouts:

1. **Drink water before, during, and after exercise:** It's essential to commence your routine well-hydrated and continue drinking water throughout your workout. After your training, make sure to consume plenty of water to replenish.

2. **Observe your urine color:** One method to measure your hydration level is to keep the color of your urine. Aim for a light golden or transparent color, indicating you are well-hydrated. Dark golden or amber-colored urine means that you need to consume more water.

3. **Drink electrolyte-rich fluids:** If you are doing strenuous exercise or sweating a lot, you may need to replenish electrolytes and fluids. Sports beverages or coconut water can be excellent choices for replenishing electrolytes.

4. **Avoid sweetened or caffeinated beverages:** beverages like cola, energy drinks, or caffeine can dehydrate you, so it's best to avoid them before and after exercise.

5. **Carry a water container with you:** Keep a water bottle with you throughout the day to remind yourself to consume water frequently.

In summation, keeping refreshed during pregnancy exercises is essential for maintaining energy levels, preventing dehydration, and supporting your developing infant. Drink water before, during, and after exercise, monitor your urine colour, drink electrolyte-rich fluids as required, avoid sweetened or stimulating beverages, and bring a water container. Following these measures allows you to remain moisturized and healthy throughout your pregnancy.

Avoid retaining your breath:

Holding your breath during activity is not recommended during pregnancy. It can cause a transient increase in blood pressure and decrease the quantity of oxygen accessible to you and your infant. Here are some strategies for preventing retaining your breath during maternity workouts:

1. **Breathe naturally:** Try to breathe naturally, repetitively throughout your exercise. Inhale through your nostrils and release through your mouth.

2. **Release during exertion:** When you are undertaking a challenging activity, release during the exertion period (e.g. when you lift the weight). This can help you maintain a consistent breathing pattern and prevent retaining your breath.

3. **Use the talk test:** A straightforward

method to measure your respiration during activity is to use the conversation test. If you can communicate in complete sentences while exercising, you are breathing appropriately. If you struggle to share or can only speak in brief sentences, you may retain your breath.

4. **Practice mindfulness:** Mindfulness strategies, such as deep breathing and meditation, can help you remain concentrated on your breath during activity and prevent retaining your breath.

In summation, retaining your breath during activity is not recommended during pregnancy. Try to breathe naturally, release during exercise, use the conversation test to observe your breathing, and practice concentration strategies to remain concentrated on your breath. By following these guidelines, you can maintain a secure and efficient exercise regimen during pregnancy.

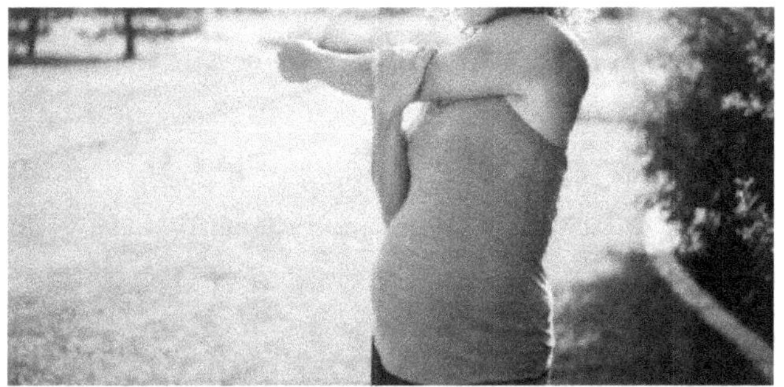

Stretching and yoga can be excellent exercises during the first trimester of pregnancy. These moderate exercises can help improve flexibility, reduce stress, and ease typical pregnancy discomforts such as back pain and muscular tightness.

However, it's essential to choose a yoga practice mainly intended for pregnancy or to work with a qualified pregnant yoga instructor, as some yoga postures may be dangerous during pregnancy.

During the first trimester, it's essential to avoid any positions that require laying on your stomach or back for a prolonged amount of time, as this can decrease the oxygen supply to your infant. It's also essential to prevent profound rotating movements, as these can stretch your abdominal muscles and place pressure on your cervix.

Instead, concentrate on moderate stretches and yoga postures for pregnancy, such as standing poses, hip openers, and delicate forward bends. These postures can help alleviate tightness in the body, increase circulation, and encourage tranquillity.

It's essential to listen to your body during yoga and stretching and to avoid exerting yourself too hard. If you experience pain or irritation, immediately cease the position and communicate with your healthcare practitioner.

Flexibility and yoga can be excellent ways to support your health and well-being during the first trimester of pregnancy, as long as you choose safe and appropriate postures and respond to your body's requirements.

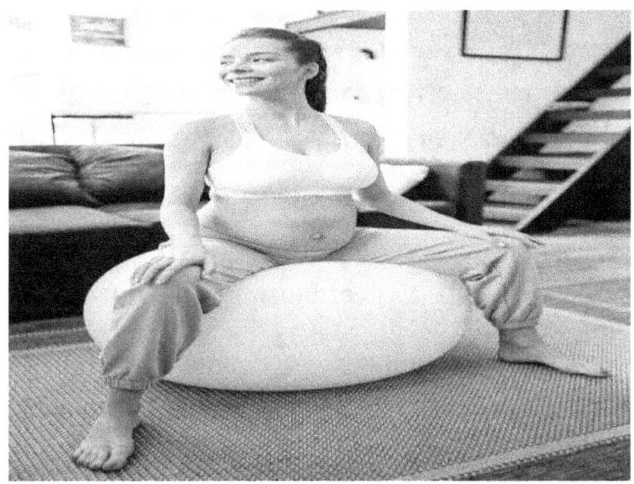

Pelvic floor movements, also known as Kegels, can be an essential component of your fitness regimen during the first trimester of pregnancy. These movements help strengthen the muscles that support the bladder, uterus, and intestines, which can help decrease the risk of incontinence and other pelvic floor disorders.

To execute pelvic floor movements:

Merely constrict and hold the muscles around your vagina and anus as if attempting to halt urine passage.

Hold the contraction for a few seconds, then release and soften the muscles.

Repeat this exercise several times throughout the day, progressively increasing the duration of the contraction as your muscles become more robust.

It's essential to be conscious of your respiration during pelvic floor movements and to prevent retaining your breath or tensing other muscles.

Pelvic floor movements are safe and efficient during pregnancy and can be practiced throughout all three trimesters. However, avoiding overexerting your pelvic floor muscles is essential, as this can contribute to muscular tension and damage. Speak with your healthcare practitioner or a physical therapist if you have any inquiries about conducting pelvic floor movements securely and successfully during pregnancy.

CHAPTER THREE

Second Trimester Workouts

The second trimester of pregnancy is often referred to as the "golden period" of pregnancy, as many women begin to feel more vitality and experience fewer pregnancy symptoms. This can be an excellent time to concentrate on maintaining your fitness and preparing your body for childbearing.

During the second trimester, listening to your body and modifying your exercise regimen as required is essential. Your body is more flexible, and your equilibrium has improved, enabling you to increase the intensity and duration of your exercises comfortably.

In this portion of the program, we will examine different fitness choices that are safe and effective during the second trimester, including cardiovascular exercises such as swimming and pregnancy callisthenics, as well as strength training exercises that can help maintain muscle tone and prevent damage. It's essential to consult with your healthcare practitioner before beginning any exercise regimen during pregnancy, listen to your body, and make modifications as required.

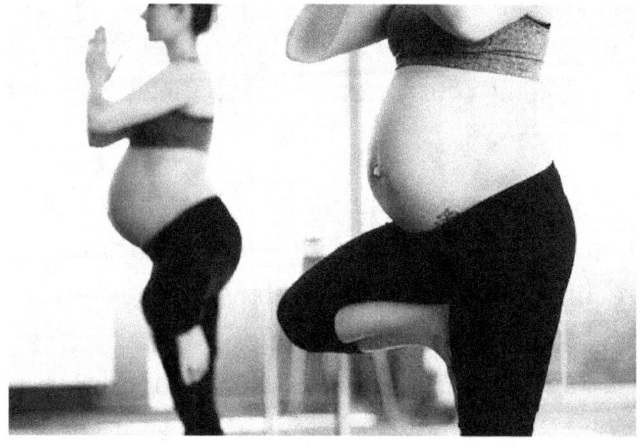

Cardiovascular activities can be an excellent method to maintain your fitness and support cardiovascular health during the second trimester of pregnancy. Some safe and efficient cardiovascular activities for the second trimester include:

1. **Swimming:** Swimming is a low-impact activity that can help increase cardiovascular endurance and strengthen your limbs, thighs, and back muscles. It's also wonderful to remain calm and alleviate joint discomfort during the sweltering summer months.

2. **Walking:** Walking is a low-impact activity that can be done almost anywhere and requires no specific apparatus. It can help increase cardiovascular endurance and strengthen your thighs and pelvis muscles.

3. **Prenatal exercises:** Prenatal aerobics courses are intended mainly for pregnant women and can be enjoyable and efficient in increasing cardiovascular endurance and maintaining fitness during pregnancy. These courses generally include a combination of low-impact activities, such as swaying and marching, and strength training exercises.

4.   **Stationary pedalling:** Stationary cycling can be a safe and efficient method to increase cardiovascular fitness during pregnancy, as it is low-impact and enables you to regulate the intensity of your exercise. Just modify the saddle and handlebars to suit your shifting frame, and avoid standing up on the pedals or pedalling at a high intensity.

It's essential to attend to your body during cardiopulmonary activity and prevent straining yourself too hard. Be careful to remain refreshed, take pauses as required, and avoid activities involving abrupt movements or direction changes. If you experience pain or irritation, immediately cease the exercise and communicate with your healthcare practitioner.

Strength training can be essential to your second-trimester exercise regimen, as it can help maintain muscle tone and prevent damage. However, it's necessary to use prudence and modify your regimen as your body changes during pregnancy.

Here are some suggestions for safe and efficient exercise training during the second trimester:

1. **Use lighter weights:** As your body changes and your Centre of gravity alters, using smaller weights and concentrating on high repetitions is essential. This will help you maintain a muscular tone without placing an excessive burden on your joints.

2.   **Avoid activities that place pressure on your midsection:** activities that require you to lay on your back or put pressure on your abdomen, such as crunches and sit-ups, should be avoided after the first trimester. Instead, concentrate on movements that activate your core, such as pelvis tilts and modified planks.

3.   **Incorporate bodyweight exercises:** Bodyweight exercises, such as squats and lunges, can efficiently maintain muscular tone without the need for apparatus. Just be sure to use the correct technique and prevent overexerting yourself.

4.   **Focus on balance and stability:** As your body transforms during pregnancy, your equilibrium and peace may be impacted. Incorporating activities that concentrate on credit, such as single-leg deadlifts and modified yoga postures, can help strengthen your balance and prevent

accidents.

It's essential to communicate with your healthcare practitioner before beginning any strength training regimen during pregnancy, and to listen to your body and make modifications as required. Remember to remain refreshed, pause as needed, and avoid retaining your breath while raising weights. If you experience pain or irritation, immediately cease the activity and communicate with your healthcare practitioner.

Stretching and yoga in the Second Trimester Workouts

Stretching and yoga can be advantageous to your second-trimester exercise regimen. These movements can help increase flexibility, decrease muscular tightness, and alleviate stress.

Here are some suggestions for safe and efficient

flexibility and yoga during the second trimester:

1. **Focus on delicate stretches:** As your body transforms during pregnancy, focusing on gentle exercises that don't place excessive stress on your joints is essential. Avoid overstretching and respond to your body.

2. **Avoid deep twists and backbends:** They should be avoided during pregnancy, as they can pressure your abdominal and vaginal region. Instead, concentrate on positions that free up the torso and pelvis.

3. **Use objects for support:** entities such as blocks, blankets, and harnesses can provide additional support and help you adjust positions as required.

4. **Avoid heated yoga:** heated yoga can increase your body temperature and

potentially damage your infant. Stick to standard temperature yoga sessions.

5. **Incorporate pelvic floor exercises:** Pelvic floor exercises can be incorporated into your yoga practice to help strengthen the muscles that support your genital organs.

It's essential to consult with your healthcare practitioner before beginning any new exercise regimen during pregnancy, including flexibility and yoga. Listen to your body, pause as required, and avoid overexerting yourself. If you experience pain or irritation, immediately cease the activity and communicate with your healthcare practitioner.

Pelvic floor movements in the Second Trimester Workouts

Pelvic floor movements, or Kegels, are essential to your second-trimester fitness regimen. These movements help strengthen the muscles that support your pelvic organs, which can help decrease the chance of bladder incontinence and other pelvic floor disorders.

Here are some suggestions for safe and efficient pelvic floor movements during the second trimester:

1. **Find the correct muscles:** To do Kegels, you must recognize the muscles that regulate continence. To do this, consider preventing the discharge of urine when you're in the bathroom. The muscles you use to do this are your pelvic floor muscles.

2. **Start slowly:** Begin by constricting your pelvic floor muscles for 3-5 seconds, then release for 3-5 seconds. Repeat ten times, three times a day.

3. **Gradually increase the duration and intensity:** As your pelvic floor muscles get stronger, gradually increase the duration and intensity of your Kegels. Try contracting your muscles for 10 seconds or doing more repetitions.

4. **Incorporate Kegels into your exercise routine:** You can do Kegels while sitting, standing, or lying down. Try incorporating them into your yoga or strength training regimen.

5. **Be consistent:** Consistency is essential when it comes to Kegels. Aim to do them daily, and be diligent as you work to strengthen your pelvic floor muscles.

It's essential to consult with your healthcare practitioner before beginning any new exercise regimen during pregnancy, including pelvic floor movements. Listen to your body, pause as required, and avoid overexerting yourself. If you experience pain or irritation, immediately cease the activity and communicate with your healthcare practitioner.

CHAPTER FOUR

Third Trimester Workouts

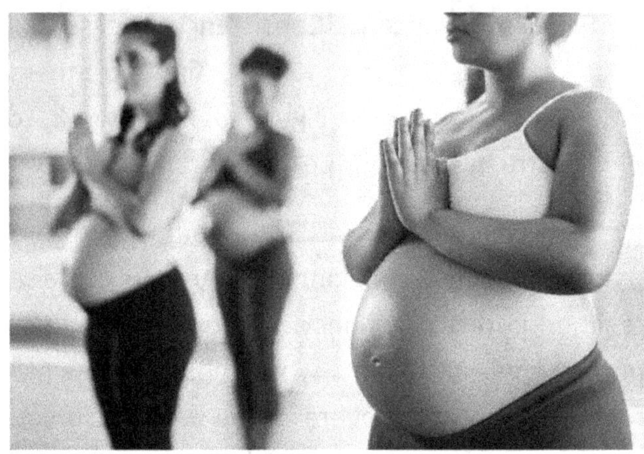

The third trimester of pregnancy can be physically challenging, but maintaining a regular exercise regimen can help prepare your body for labour and delivery and lessen typical pregnancy-related discomforts. However, it's essential to modify your exercise regimen to accommodate your shifting body and prevent placing excessive stress on yourself and your infant.

Here are some general guidelines for safe and efficient third-trimester workouts:

1. Focus on low-impact activities: High-impact exercises like sprinting and leaping can be uncomfortable and potentially dangerous as your abdomen develops. Instead, concentrate on low-impact activities like strolling, swimming, and pregnant yoga.

2. **Adjust strength training exercises:** If you're still incorporating strength training into your regimen, be sure to modify activities to prevent placing tension on your abdominal muscles. Avoid crunches and splits, and opt for exercises like squats and lunges that engage your lower body.

3. **Pay attention to your body:** As you approach your due date, attending to your body and modifying your exercise regimen as required is essential. If you experience

pain or irritation, immediately cease the activity and communicate with your healthcare practitioner.

4. **Stay moistened:** As always, staying refreshed during your exercises is essential. Drink plenty of water before, during, and after activity to prevent dehydration.

5. **Consider joining a pregnancy exercise class:** pregnancy exercise programs can provide an encouraging and secure environment for pregnant women to exercise. Look for courses for the third trimester or programs incorporating movements to prepare your body for labour and delivery.

Remember, it's essential to consult with your healthcare practitioner before beginning any new exercise regimen during pregnancy, particularly in the third trimester. They can help you determine certain appropriate activities for you and your infant.

Cardiovascular activities In the Third Trimester

Workouts

Cardiovascular activities In the Third Trimester Workouts

Cardiopulmonary exercises can still be an essential part of your fitness regimen during the third trimester. Still, choosing low-impact exercises that are gentle on your body and prevent placing excessive stress on your infant is essential.

Here are some safe cardiovascular activities to consider during the third trimester:

1. **Walking:** Walking is a low-impact activity that can help you maintain your cardiovascular health without burdening your joints. Try to stroll for at least 30 minutes daily, and consider splitting up your outings into shorter segments if necessary.

2.   **Swimming:** Swimming is a beautiful method to get cardiovascular activity while keeping pressure off your joints. Consider swimming loops or attending a water exercise session to increase your pulse rate.

3.   **Stationary pedalling:** Stationary cycling can be a safe and efficient method to increase your pulse rate during the third trimester. Be careful to change the bench height to accommodate your expanding abdomen and prevent placing excessive stress on your lower back.

4.   **Elliptical trainer:** An elliptical trainer can provide a low-impact cardiovascular exercise while exercising your upper and lower body. Be sure to choose a machine with handlebars to help you maintain your equilibrium and prevent collapsing.

5.   **Low-impact aerobics classes:** Consider attending a low-impact exercise class mainly for pregnant women to get their pulse rate up and remain active.

Remember, listening to your body and preventing straining yourself too hard during the third trimester is essential. If you experience pain or irritation, immediately cease the activity and communicate with your healthcare practitioner.

Strength conditioning In the Third Trimester Workouts

Strength training can still be a valuable part of your exercise regimen during the third trimester. Still, it's essential to make some modifications to guarantee your and your infant's safety. Here are some suggestions for physical exercise during the third trimester:

1.   **Use smaller weights:** As your infant develops, you may discover that you need

to decrease the weight you raise. Choose consequences that are comfortable and don't burden your body.

2.   **Focus on form:** During the third trimester, your body may be more susceptible to injury, so it's essential to focus on correct form and technique when conducting strength training activities. Consider working with a teacher who has experience with pregnancy exercise.

3.   **Avoid activities that put pressure on your abdomen:** exercises that require you to lay on your back, such as chest press, should be avoided during the third trimester as they can place pressure on your uterus and impact the blood supply to your infant.

4.   **Incorporate body weight activities:** Bodyweight exercises can safely and efficiently develop strength during the third trimester. Consider activities such as

squats, lunges, and modified push-ups.

5.   **Take pauses as needed:** During the third trimester, your body may become exhausted more readily. Be careful to pause as required and respond to your body's indications.

Remember, it's essential to consult with your healthcare practitioner before beginning any new physical exercise regimen during pregnancy. They can provide instructions on what kinds of activities are secure for you and your infant.

Stretching and Pilates in the Third Trimester Workouts

During the third trimester, stretching and yoga can help maintain flexibility, decrease discomfort, and prepare your body for childbirth. However, it's essential to modify your regimen as your body changes. Here are some suggestions for flexibility and exercise during the third trimester:

1. **Focus on delicate stretching:** During the third trimester, your ligaments and joints may become more loosened and prone to injury. Focus on gradual extension rather than straining your body to the maximum. Aim to lengthen significant muscular groups such as your pelvis, back, and thighs.

2. **Avoid deep twists and forward bends:** As your abdomen develops, it's essential to avoid deep twists and turns that can constrict your uterine and restrict blood supply to your infant. Instead, concentrate on moderate rotations and adjusted postures that support your abdomen.

3. **Use props:** Props such as blocks, blankets, and harnesses can help you change positions and make them more

comfortable. For example, use a partnership to support your pelvis in a sitting forward fold or a harness to assist you in reaching your feet in a seated forward bend.

4. **Practice pelvic floor exercises:** The third trimester is a good time to concentrate on pelvic floor exercises, which can help prepare your body for childbirth and prevent incontinence. Incorporate movements such as Kegels into your stretching and yoga practice.

5. **Listen to your body:** As always, listening to your body and adjusting your regimen as required is essential. If a posture feels uncomfortable or excruciating, abandon it and continue to another pose.

Remember, it's essential to consult with your healthcare practitioner before beginning any new stretching or yoga practice during pregnancy.

They can provide instructions on secure positions for you and your infant.

Pelvic floor movements In the Third Trimester

Workouts

Pelvic floor movements, also known as Kegels, are essential throughout pregnancy but can be particularly advantageous during the third trimester as you prepare for childbirth. Here are some suggestions for pelvic floor movements during the third trimester:

1. Find the correct muscles: To do pelvic floor movements, you need to compress and release the muscles in your pelvic floor. To locate these muscles, try blocking the passage of urine midstream. The muscles you use to do this are your pelvic floor muscles.

2. **Practice regularly:** Aim to do pelvic floor movements every day, preferably several times daily. Start with a few repetitions

and eventually build up to 10 repetitions per session.

3. **Incorporate into everyday activities:** You can do pelvic floor movements anytime. Try doing them while sitting at your workstation, standing in line, or watching TV.

4. **Change as needed:** As your pregnancy progresses, you may need to change your pelvic floor movements. For example, you may need to do them sitting or lying down as your abdomen develops.

5. **Seek guidance:** If you need to know if you're doing pelvic floor movements appropriately or have any questions about your pelvic floor health, consult your healthcare practitioner. If required, they can assist and recommend you to a pelvic floor physical therapist.

Remember, pelvic floor movements can help prevent incontinence and other pelvic floor problems during and after pregnancy, but they are not a replacement for medical treatment. Speak with your healthcare practitioner if you have any questions about your pelvic floor health.

CHAPTER FIVE

Nutrition and Hydration

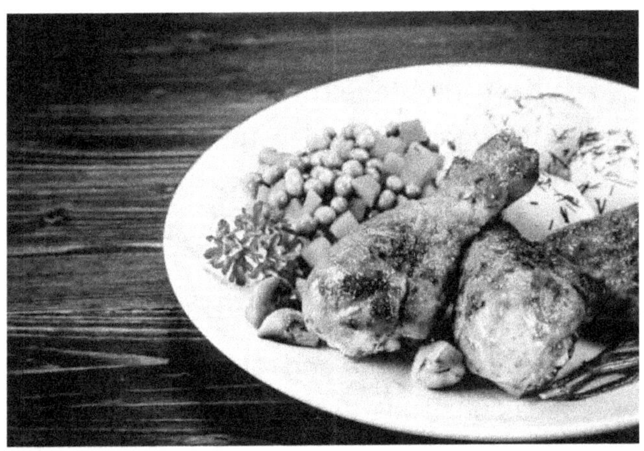

Nutrition and hydration are essential components of a successful pregnancy. Eating a balanced diet and keeping refreshed can help support the growth and development of your infant, as well as help you feel your best. Here are some suggestions for nourishment and hydration during pregnancy:

- **Eat nutrient-rich foods:** Eat a balanced

diet with mixed fruits, vegetables, whole cereals, lean proteins, and healthy lipids. These meals provide essential nutrients like folic acid, calcium, and omega-3 fatty acids.

- **Keep moistened:** Drink plenty of water throughout the day to keep refreshed. Aim for at least 8-10 glasses of water daily, and more if you exercise or in humid conditions.

- **Limit caffeine and alcohol:** Too much caffeine and alcohol can harm your infant. Limit caffeine consumption to no more than 200 milligrams per day, and eliminate drinking completely.

- **Consider taking a prenatal vitamin:** Prenatal supplements can help ensure you receive all the nutrition you need for a healthy pregnancy, including folic acid, iron, and calcium.

- **Listen to your body:** Your body may have different nutritional requirements during pregnancy, so it's essential to listen to your body and consume when you're famished. Don't stress too much about calorie tracking - concentrate on finishing a selection of nutritious meals and keeping refreshed.

Remember to communicate with your healthcare practitioner if you have any inquiries or concerns about your nutrition or hydration during pregnancy. They can provide individualized recommendations based on your particular requirements and health background.

Importance of adequate nourishment

Proper nourishment during pregnancy is essential for both the mother's health and the infant's growth and development. Here are some explanations of why:

1. **Supports healthy prenatal development:** Proper nourishment provides essential nutrients that support healthy embryonic growth and development, including folic acid, iron, and omega-3 fatty acids.

2. **Reduces the chance of birth abnormalities:** Folic acid is essential during the first trimester of pregnancy, as it can help reduce the risk of neural tube malformations.

3. **Supports maternal health:** Proper nourishment during pregnancy can also help support the mother's health, lowering the chance of complications like anaemia, gestational diabetes, and pre-eclampsia.

4. **Supports breastfeeding:** A nutritious diet during pregnancy can also help support successful breastfeeding after the

infant is delivered.

5. **Establishes healthy habits:** Pregnancy is a beautiful time to establish healthy dietary habits that can continue into subsequent life, helping to support long-term health and well-being.

It's essential to note that every woman's nutritional demands during pregnancy may differ, so you must communicate with your healthcare practitioner about your particular needs and dietary requirements.

They can provide individualized recommendations based on your unique health background and underlying medical conditions.

Nutrient requirements during pregnancy

During pregnancy, a woman's nutritional

requirements increase to support the growth and development of the infant. Here are some of the essential nutrients that are particularly important during pregnancy:

1. **Folic acid:** Folic acid is essential for normal neural tube development in the embryo, specifically during the first trimester. Women expecting or intending to become pregnant should take a daily multivitamin containing 400-800 milligrams of folic acid.

2. **Iron:** Iron is essential for generating red blood cells and transporting oxygen to the embryo. Pregnant women require more iron than non-pregnant women and may need an iron supplement if their iron levels are insufficient.

3. **Calcium:** Calcium is essential for the development of the baby's bones and teeth and the mother's bone health.

Pregnant women are recommended to consume 1000-1300 milligrams of calcium daily.

4. **Vitamin D:** Vitamin D helps the body assimilate calcium and is essential for bone health. Pregnant women are recommended to consume 600-800 international units (IU) of vitamin D daily.

5. **Omega-3 fatty acids:** Omega-3 fatty acids are essential for embryonic brain and ocular development. Pregnant women must consume at least 200-300 milligrams of omega-3 fatty acids daily.

6. **Protein:** Protein is essential for embryonic growth and development and the mother's own muscle healing and growth. Pregnant women are recommended to consume 25 grams of protein daily.

It's essential to note that every woman's nutritional demands during pregnancy may differ, so it's vital to communicate with your healthcare practitioner about your particular needs and dietary requirements.

They can provide individualized recommendations based on your unique health background and underlying medical conditions.

Staying moisturized is essential during pregnancy to support the increased blood volume, maintain healthy placental fluid levels, and help prevent constipation and urinary tract infections. Here are some general recommendations for keeping moisturized during pregnancy:

1. **Drink plenty of water:** Aim to drink at least 8-10 glasses (64-80 ounces) of water per day, or more if you are physically

engaged or in humid conditions.

2. **Limit caffeine and sugary drinks:** Caffeine and sugary beverages can be dehydrating and should be ingested in limitation during pregnancy. Restricting caffeine consumption to 200 milligrams per day (about one 12-ounce cup of coffee) is recommended.

3. **Include water-rich foods in your diet:** Eating foods with high water content, such as fruits and vegetables, can help you remain hydrated.

4. **Pay attention to hunger cues:** If you feel parched, it's an indication that your body requires more fluids.

5. **Be cautious of fluid loss:** Vomiting, diarrhoea, and perspiration can cause fluid loss and increase the risk of

dehydration. If you experience any of these symptoms, it's essential to replenish fluids and electrolytes.

It's essential to communicate with your healthcare practitioner about your specific hydration requirements during pregnancy, particularly if you have any preexisting medical conditions or complications. They can provide individualized recommendations based on your particular health background.

Modifications for Common Pregnancy Symptoms

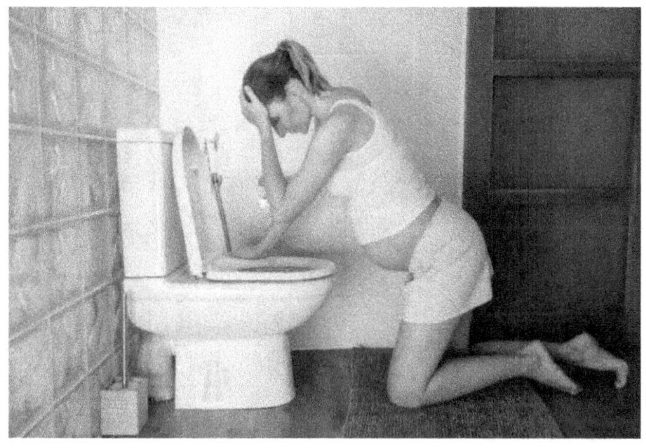

Many women experience typical symptoms during pregnancy that can impact their ability to exercise or conduct everyday activities. Here are some modifications that can help handle these symptoms:

1. **Nausea and vomiting:** Nausea and

vomiting can make exercising challenging or conducting everyday activities difficult. Eating small, frequent meals throughout the day, keeping refreshed, and avoiding intense smells or flavors can help control symptoms. Exercise during the times of day when sickness is least severe, and select moderate activities such as strolling or yoga.

2.   **Fatigue:** Fatigue is a typical complaint during pregnancy, and it can make exercise and everyday activities challenging. Try to get plenty of rest, remain refreshed, and prevent overexertion. Short, frequent bursts of exercise, such as 10-15 minutes of strolling or stretching, can help control tiredness without causing further exhaustion.

3.   **Back pain:** Back pain is frequent during pregnancy, particularly in the later phases. Avoid activities that place unnecessary

pressure on the lower back, such as deep lunges or hefty hauling. Opt for moderate activities such as pelvis tilts, wall lunges, or swimming, which can help strengthen the muscles supporting the back.

4.   **Swelling:** Swelling, specifically in the feet and ankles, is a typical complaint during pregnancy. Avoid activities that require protracted standing or reclining, and elevate the knees whenever feasible. Gentle movements like swimming or yoga can help improve circulation and minimize puffiness.

5.   **Shortness of breath:** As the uterus develops, it can press up against the diaphragm, resulting in shortness of breath. Opt for moderate activities such as strolling or yoga, and avoid movements that require retaining your breath or stressing.

It's essential to consult with your healthcare practitioner or a qualified maternal fitness professional before beginning any exercise program during pregnancy, particularly if you are experiencing any of these symptoms. They can provide individualized recommendations and modifications based on your health background and exercise level.

Nausea and vomiting are typical sensations many women encounter during pregnancy, particularly in the first trimester. Numerous factors, including endocrine changes, heightened amounts of stress, and changes in the intestinal system, can trigger these symptoms. However, some modifications can help ease these symptoms and enable pregnant women to continue their exercise regimen.

1. **Timing:** Exercising in the morning or before meals may help prevent sickness and vomiting, as a full stomach can

provoke these symptoms.

2.   **Hydration:** Staying refreshed before, during, and after exercise can help prevent dehydration, which can exacerbate sickness and vomiting. Sipping water or nutritional beverages during activity may be beneficial.

3.   **Intensity:** Lowering the intensity of the activity or participating in low-impact activities such as strolling, swimming, or yoga can help alleviate sickness and vomiting.

4.   **Acupressure:** Applying pressure to particular places on the body, such as the wrist, may help alleviate sickness and regurgitation. Wearing acupressure bracelets on the forearms during activity may be beneficial.

5. **Consult with a healthcare provider:** If sickness and vomiting are intense and continuous, it is essential to consult with a healthcare provider to ensure that no underlying medical conditions require treatment.

Fatigue

Fatigue is a typical complaint encountered by many women during pregnancy, particularly in the first and third trimesters. It is often triggered by endocrine changes, heightened stress, and alterations in the body's metabolism. However, there are some modifications that can help alleviate exhaustion and enable pregnant women to continue their exercise regimen.

1. **Rest:** Taking pauses and incorporating rest intervals during exercises can help prevent unnecessary exhaustion.

2. **Hydration:** Staying refreshed before, during, and after exercise can help

prevent dehydration, which can exacerbate tiredness.

3.   **Intensity:** Lowering the intensity of the activity or participating in low-impact activities such as strolling, swimming, or yoga can help alleviate exhaustion.

4.   **Timing:** Exercising when you feel most energetic, such as in the morning or after sleep, can help prevent unnecessary exhaustion.

5.   **Consult with a healthcare provider:** If exhaustion is extreme and continuous, it is essential to consult with a healthcare provider to ensure that no underlying medical conditions require treatment.

Back discomfort is a typical pregnancy complaint, particularly in the later phases. It is often caused by increased weight and pressure on the lower back and pelvis. However, some modifications can help alleviate back discomfort and enable pregnant women to continue their exercise regimen.

1. **Proper alignment:** Maintaining excellent balance during exercises can help minimize pressure on the back muscles.

2. **Supportive gear:** Wearing supportive sneakers and a supportive waistband or belt during exercises can help alleviate pressure on the lower back.

3. **Low-impact activities:** Doing low-impact exercises such as swimming or yoga can help alleviate back discomfort.

4. **Core strengthening:** Strengthening the core muscles can help alleviate back discomfort by providing more fantastic support to the vertebrae.

5. **Consult with a healthcare provider:** If back pain is significant and continuous, it is essential to consult with a healthcare provider to ensure that no underlying medical conditions require treatment.

Swelling and varicose veins

Swelling and varicose veins are typical pregnancy symptoms that can make exercising uncomfortable. Here are some modifications that can help alleviate these symptoms:

1. **Stay moistened:** Staying hydrated can help minimize puffiness.

2.   **Avoid standing or sitting for lengthy periods:** Standing or sitting for prolonged periods can exacerbate puffiness and increase the risk of varicose veins. Try to take numerous pauses and walk around frequently.

3.   **Wear compression pantyhose:** Compression stockings can help increase blood flow and decrease puffiness and irritation in the thighs.

4.   **Elevate your legs:** Elevating your ankles above your torso for 20 minutes a few times daily can help decrease puffiness.

5.   **Low-impact activities:** Low-impact exercises such as strolling, swimming, and pedalling can help increase circulation and decrease puffiness.

6.   **Consult with a healthcare provider:** If

puffiness or varicose veins are significant or excruciating, it is essential to consult with a healthcare provider to ensure that no underlying medical conditions require treatment.

Shortness of respiration

Shortness of breath is a typical sensation during pregnancy as the developing embryo places pressure on the diaphragm and airways. Here are some modifications that can help alleviate this symptom:

1. **Slow down:** Try to slow down your speed and take more frequent pauses during exercise.

2. **Focus on breathing:** Take deliberate, deep breaths during activity and focus on releasing completely to help increase oxygen consumption.

3. **Modify exercise intensity:** Reduce the

intensity of your exercises to prevent overexertion, which can exacerbate shortness of breath.

4. **Maintain excellent alignment:** excellent posture can help free up the thorax and enhance respiration.

5. **Try activities that promote relaxation:** Gentle exercises such as yoga, stretching, and meditation can help decrease tension and promote peace, which can help alleviate shortness of breath.

6. **Consult with a healthcare provider:** If shortness of breath is significant or continuous, it is essential to consult with a healthcare provider to ensure that no underlying medical conditions require treatment.

Pelvic Floor Health

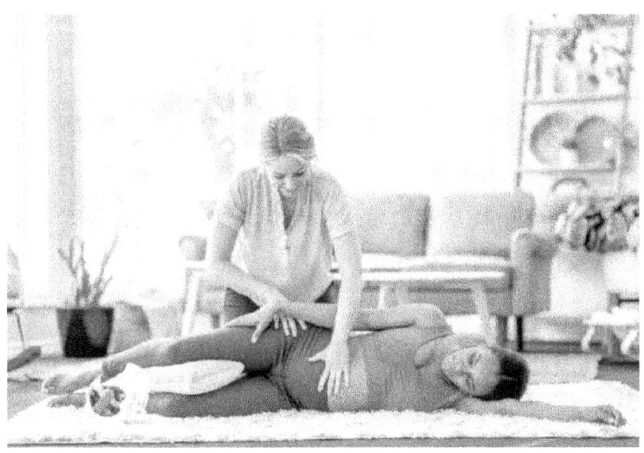

The pelvic floor is a collection of muscles that create a sling-like structure at the root of the pelvis. These muscles are responsible for maintaining the pelvic structures such as the bladder, uterus, and rectum. During childbearing, the pelvic floor muscles experience substantial alterations and can become compromised or injured. This can contribute to bladder incontinence, pelvic organ collapse, and sexual dysfunction. Therefore, maintaining excellent pelvic floor health during and after childbearing is vital for general well-being.

The pelvic floor is essential during pregnancy as it supports the developing uterus and helps regulate urinary and digestive function. As the uterus develops during pregnancy, it can place pressure on the pelvic floor muscles, which can contribute to compromised or injured muscles. This can create difficulties such as bladder incontinence, faecal incontinence, and pelvic organ collapse.

In addition, the pelvic floor muscles play a critical part during childbirth by forcing the infant out. Strengthening the pelvic floor muscles during pregnancy can help prepare them for this challenge and may decrease the risk of complications during delivery, such as ripping or episiotomy.

After childbearing, the pelvic floor muscles may become further compromised, making it challenging to regulate urinary and stool function. This can also impact reproductive performance and general quality of life. Therefore, maintaining excellent pelvic floor health during pregnancy can help decrease the chance of these conditions and support general well-being.

Exercises for pelvic floor strength and relaxation

There are a variety of activities that can help increase pelvic floor strength and relaxation during pregnancy. These activities include:

1. **Kegels:** Kegels are a form of exercise that includes constricting and releasing the pelvic floor muscles. To execute a Kegel, tighten the muscles that you would use to halt the passage of urine. Hold for a few

seconds, then release. Repeat for several repetitions throughout the day.

2.   **Squats:** Squats are excellent practice for developing pelvic floor strength. Stand with your ankles shoulder-width apart and lower yourself into a crouching position as if you were reclining in a chair. Make careful to maintain your spine straight and your knees over your ankles. Hold for a few seconds, then ascend back up.

3.   **Bridges:** Bridges are another excellent practice for the pelvic floor. Lie on your back with your knees bowed and your feet level on the floor. Raise your pelvis toward the ceiling, tightening your buttocks and activating your pelvic floor muscles. Hold for a few seconds, then lower back down.

4.   **Pelvic tilts:** Pelvic tilts are a reasonable practice that can help enhance pelvic floor relaxation. Lie on your back with your

knees bowed and your feet level on the floor. Slowly rotate your tailbone forward and rearward, maintaining your lower back on the floor.

5.   Deep breathing techniques can also help promote pelvic floor relaxation. Take deliberate, steady breaths, breathing through your nostrils and releasing through your mouth. As you live, concentrate on releasing your pelvic floor muscles.

Speaking to your healthcare practitioner before beginning any new exercise routine, particularly during pregnancy, is essential. They can assist you.

Establish which activities are secure and appropriate for you based on your requirements and health condition.

CHAPTER EIGHT

Postpartum Exercise

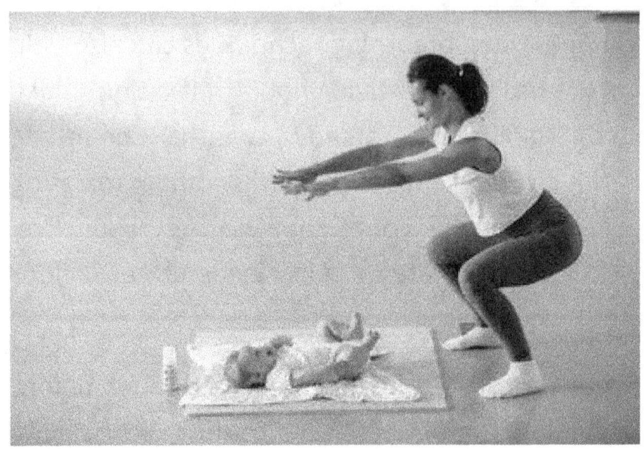

Postpartum exercise refers to physical activity conducted by women after giving birth to help them recuperate from childbearing and reclaim their pre-pregnancy strength, endurance, and fitness levels. Postpartum exercise can assist new mothers physiologically and spiritually, and it can also aid in managing postpartum melancholy, anxiety, and tension.

It's essential to note that postpartum exercise should only be undertaken after permission from a healthcare practitioner, as the scheduling and intensity of the activity will depend on the type of delivery and individual health condition. In general, it's recommended that women delay at least six weeks after natural delivery and eight weeks after surgical delivery before starting exercise. Additionally, new mothers should commence with moderate movements and progressively increase intensity and endurance as they feel comfortable and their body permits.

Benefits of postpartum exercise

Postpartum exercise has several advantages, including:

1. **Restoring physical function:** After delivery, the body experiences several changes, including endocrine changes, loss of muscular strength, and muscle and joint stiffness. Postpartum exercise can

help recover physical performance by strengthening the muscles, increasing flexibility, and decreasing discomfort.

2. **Reducing the chance of postpartum depression:** Exercise has been shown to produce neurotransmitters and natural mood enhancers. Regular exercise can help decrease the likelihood of postpartum melancholy and enhance general mental health.

3. **Improving cardiovascular health:** Postpartum exercise can help improve cardiovascular health by increasing heart rate and improving blood flow.

4. **Helping with weight loss:** Exercise can help women shed pregnancy weight and enhance body composition by decreasing body fat and increasing lean muscle mass.

5. **Boosting energy levels:** Many new mothers experience exhaustion and reduced energy levels after delivery. Exercise can help increase energy levels by enhancing circulation, increasing oxygen distribution to the body, and producing neurotransmitters.

6. **Strengthening pelvic floor muscles:** The pelvic floor muscles may become compromised during pregnancy and childbirth, leading to problems such as incontinence. Postpartum activity can help strengthen these muscles and enhance general reproductive health.

Postpartum exercise can help new mothers feel more invigorated, decrease the chance of postpartum melancholy, and enhance physical performance and public health.

It is recommended to wait until after the six-week postpartum examination before beginning any exercise regimen. However, listening to your body and pressing yourself slowly is essential. Some women may need to delay longer depending on the sort of childbirth and any complications. It is recommended to consult with your healthcare practitioner before commencing any postpartum exercise regimen.

Safe childbirth activities

Safe postpartum activities generally depend on variables such as the type of delivery, the recuperation process, and the degree of fitness before and during pregnancy. However, some safe postpartum activities that new mothers can commence with include:

1. **Walking:** Walking is a low-impact activity that can help improve circulation, strengthen the muscles, and improve general fitness. New mothers can begin with brief walks around the house or neighborhood and progressively increase the duration and intensity of the walks.

2. **Pelvic floor exercises:** Strengthening the pelvic floor muscles after childbearing can help prevent incontinence and encourage recovery. Kegel movements are a straightforward and efficient method to strengthen the pelvic floor muscles.

3. Yoga can help increase flexibility, equilibrium, and tranquillity. Postpartum yoga courses tailored for new mothers can help target particular regions of the body that may be impacted by childbirth.

4. **Low-impact aerobics:** Low-impact

aerobics can help increase cardiovascular fitness without burdening the joints. New mothers can start with uncomplicated activities such as marching in place, side steps, and arm rotations and eventually graduate to more strenuous routines.

5.   **Abdominal activities:** Abdominal exercises such as pelvic tilts and moderate abdominal crunches can help strengthen the abdominal muscles and encourage recovery. However, new mothers should avoid any actions that produce soreness or irritation in the abdominal region.

It is essential to communicate with a healthcare practitioner before beginning any postpartum exercise regimen to ensure that it is safe and appropriate for the individual's particular requirements and rehabilitation process.

CHAPTER NINE

Exercise Safety Considerations

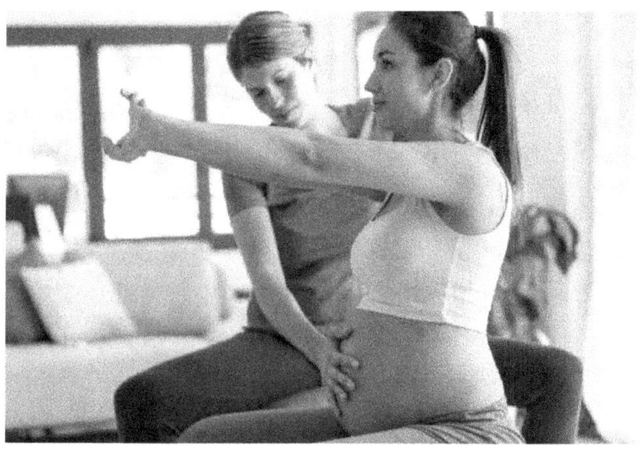

Exercise safety considerations are crucial in any exercise program but become even more essential during pregnancy and childbirth. It is critical to prioritize safety to guarantee both the mother's and the baby's health and well-being.

The following are some exercise safety considerations to bear in mind during pregnancy and postpartum:

1. Consult with your healthcare practitioner before beginning or completing any exercise regimen.

2. Listen to your body and cease practising if you experience discomfort, confusion, or shortness of breath.

3. Avoid high-impact movements and activities that involve a risk of collapsing or physical sports.

4. Use correct posture and technique during activities to prevent damage.

5. Avoid activities that involve laying on your back after the first trimester of pregnancy.

6. Stay refreshed and avoid practising in

sweltering circumstances.

7. Gradually increase the intensity and duration of exercise to prevent overexertion.

8. Incorporate leisure days into your exercise regimen to enable your body to recuperate.

9. Avoid activities that pressure the pelvic floor muscles postpartum.

10. Consider working with a certified pregnancy or postpartum exercise professional who can provide individualized direction and support.

While exercise during pregnancy is typically safe and advantageous, it's essential to be conscious of caution signals indicating you should cease exercising and seek medical treatment. These caution signals include:

1. Vaginal haemorrhage or discolouration

2. Contractions that continue after relaxation or occur more than four times in an hour

3. Dizziness or faintness

4. Shortness of breath before exercise

5. Chest discomfort

6. Headache that continues after relaxation or intensifies in intensity

7. Muscle stiffness or difficulty walking

8. Calf discomfort or thickening

If you experience any of these caution signals while exercising during pregnancy, cease immediately and seek medical treatment. Speaking to your healthcare practitioner before commencing any exercise program during pregnancy is essential to ensure it's safe for you and your infant.

Precautions for high-risk pregnancies

High-risk pregnancies require specific considerations when it comes to exercise. Here are some references to bear in mind:

1. **Consult with your healthcare practitioner:** Women with high-risk pregnancies should consult their healthcare provider before beginning any exercise regimen.

2. **Avoid certain activities:** Some exercises can increase the risk of damage or complications for women with high-risk pregnancies. These may include high-impact activities, exercises that require laying on your back after the first trimester, and exercises that cause unnecessary pressure on the pelvic floor.

3. **Measure your heart rate and breathing:** Women with high-risk pregnancies should measure their heart rate and respiration during activity to ensure they are not overexerting themselves.

4. **Keep moistened:** It is essential to stay refreshed during activity, particularly for

women with high-risk pregnancies.

5.   **Take numerous pauses:** Women with high-risk pregnancies should take frequent breaks during activity to prevent exhaustion.

6.   **Avoid hyperthermia:** Women with high-risk pregnancies should avoid exercising in muggy and steamy surroundings, as this can contribute to dehydration and overheating.

7.   **Listen to your body:** It is essential to stop practising if you experience any difficulty or soreness.

Remember, protecting you and your infant is essential during exercise, particularly if you have a high-risk pregnancy.

Choosing the correct fitness attire is essential to guarantee comfort, safety, and optimum performance during exercise. This is particularly essential during pregnancy, as the body is experiencing significant changes and may require different kinds of garments and equipment. Here are some guidelines for selecting the proper exercise apparel during pregnancy:

1. **Invest in a comfortable sports bra:** During pregnancy, the breasts become more significant and heavier, which can cause irritation and pressure on the ligaments that support them. Wearing a comfortable sports bra that fits well and provides sufficient support during exercise is essential.

2. **Choose comfortable and breathable clothing:** Look for fitness clothes that are made from breathable textiles, such as

cotton or moisture-wicking materials, to help keep you calm and relaxed during exercise. Choosing clothing that suits well and provides a complete range of motion is also essential.

3. **Consider compression clothing:** Compression clothing can help improve circulation, reduce puffiness, and support muscles and joints. This can be particularly beneficial during childbearing when the body is under additional pressure.

4. **Wear appropriate footwear:** Choose sporting sneakers that provide sufficient support and protection for your feet and any specific features you may need based on your exercise regimen. For example, if you intend to do a lot of strolling or sprinting, search for sneakers that are designed for those activities.

5. **Avoid hyperthermia:** During pregnancy, it is essential to avoid overheating during activity, as this can be hazardous for both you and your infant. Choose lightweight, breathable garments, consume plenty of water, and exercise in a cold, well-ventilated location.

By selecting the correct fitness attire during pregnancy, you can help ensure that you are comfortable, secure, and able to get the most out of your exercise regimen.

CHAPTER TEN

Conclusion

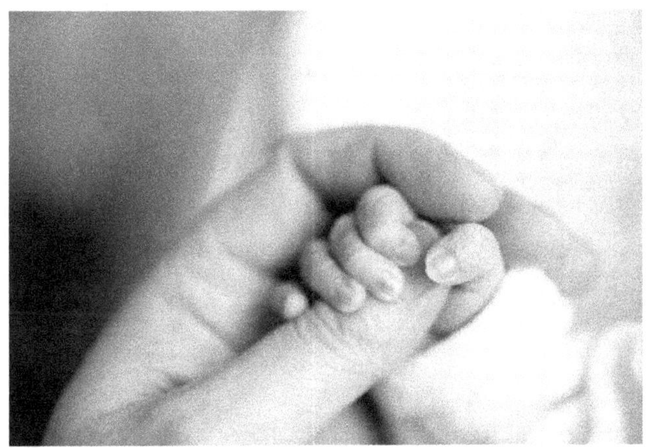

In conclusion, exercise during pregnancy is typically secure and advantageous for both the mother and the infant, provided certain precautions are taken, and a healthcare practitioner is contacted. Regular exercise can improve general health, control weight increase, alleviate pregnancy symptoms, and prepare the body for childbirth and subsequent healing.

It is essential to choose appropriate movements for each trimester, adjust routines as required for typical pregnancy complaints, and practice correct form and technique. Proper nourishment and hydration are also essential for a healthy pregnancy and should be carefully controlled.

After childbearing, postpartum exercise can help women recuperate and restore strength and fitness. It is essential to start cautiously and progressively increase the intensity of movement while paying attention to any warning signals and getting medical guidance if necessary.

Exercise safety considerations should always be considered, such as selecting the correct exercise attire and understanding caution signals to cease exercising. With appropriate precautions, exercise can be a safe and efficient way to support a healthy pregnancy and subsequent recovery.

Recap of important topics

Here is a summary of the main topics discussed in this guide:

1. First Trimester Workouts:

*   Focus on low-impact cardiovascular activities, such as strolling and swimming.

* Strength training should be modest and use the correct form and technique.

* Stretching and yoga can help decrease tension and encourage tranquillity.

* Pelvic floor movements are essential to prevent difficulties later in pregnancy.

2. Second Trimester Workouts:

* Cardiovascular activities can still be conducted but should be adjusted for comfort and safety.

* Strength exercises should be adjusted and done with smaller weights.

* Stretching and yoga can assist with flexibility and relaxation.

* Pelvic floor movements should be maintained throughout pregnancy.

3. Third Trimester Workouts:

* Low-impact cardiovascular activities such as strolling or stationary pedalling are recommended.

* Strength exercises should be ignored or adjusted to use smaller weights and fewer repetitions.

* Stretching and yoga can help decrease irritation and encourage tranquillity.

* Pelvic floor movements should continue to be done.

4. Nutrition and Hydration during Pregnancy:

* Proper nourishment is essential to support a healthy pregnancy and infant.

* Hydration recommendations include consuming at least 8-10 glasses of water daily.

* Nutrient requirements increase during pregnancy, particularly protein, iron, calcium, and folic acid.

5. Modifications for Common Pregnancy Symptoms:

* Nausea and vomiting can be alleviated with smaller, more frequent meals and avoiding triggers.

* Fatigue can be controlled with appropriate relaxation and slumber.

* Back discomfort can be alleviated with correct alignment and adjusted activities.

* Appropriate nutrition and activity modifications can decrease swelling and varicose veins.

* Shortness of breath can be controlled with appropriate breathing strategies and decreased activity.

6. Pelvic Floor Health:

* Pelvic floor movements are essential during pregnancy and after delivery to prevent difficulties such as incontinence and protrusion.

* Kegels can help strengthen the pelvic floor,

while meditative techniques can help relieve anxiety.

7. Postpartum Exercise:

* Exercise after childbearing can assist with physical and emotional rehabilitation.

* Wait until after the postpartum check-up to start exercising gently.

* Focus on low-impact activities, such as strolling or swimming, and progressively increase intensity.

8. Exercise Safety Considerations:

* Stop practising if you experience cautious symptoms like haemorrhaging or disorientation.

* High-risk pregnancies require additional precautions and communication with a healthcare practitioner.

* Proper exercise attire, such as comfortable sneakers and a supportive camisole, can help prevent injury.

Congratulations on maintaining a healthy lifestyle during pregnancy and after motherhood! Remembering postpartum exercise is secure and advantageous for both physical and emotional well-being is essential. Regular exercise can help increase energy levels, decrease tension, and assist in weight reduction.

Remember to gently and progressively increase intensity and endurance as your body permits. Be careful to listen to your body and relax when required. If you experience any soreness or irritation, cease practising and contact your healthcare practitioner.

It's also essential to prioritize self-care and create time for exercise in your everyday regimen. Whether it's taking a quick stroll, performing yoga, or doing strength training at home, locate an activity that you appreciate and suits your lifestyle.

Remember, exercise should be a component of a healthy lifestyle, not a discipline for the body. Be kind to yourself and appreciate minor successes along the road.